THE B

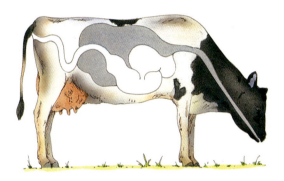

written by David Alderton
illustrated by Studio Boni/Galante,
Lorenzo Cecchi *and* Ivan Stalio

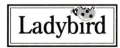

CONTENTS

	page
The Outer Body	5
The Brain and Nervous System	6
Muscles and Nerves	8
Eyes	10
Ears	12
Noses	14
Blood and The Heart	16
The Female Body	*foldout* 18-21
Animal Bodies	*foldout* 22-24
Fingers and Toes	25
Breathing	26
Tongue and Taste	28
The Digestive System	30
The Urinary System	32
Reproduction	34
Amazing Body Facts	36
Glossary	37
Index	38

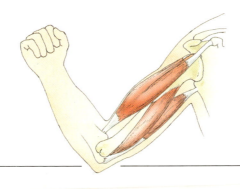

THE OUTER BODY

The outer covering of an animal's body is very important. It forms a barrier, protecting the animal from infection. Fish and reptiles have a body casing of scales. Birds have feathers which help them to fly and maintain their body temperature. Mammals have body hair, which, like feathers, traps air close to the skin and helps them to keep warm.

Hedgehogs
Hedgehogs' sharp spines are actually modified hairs. There may be 7,500 spines on an adult hedgehog's body. Newborn hedgehogs have about one hundred white spines.

Frogs, newts and toads
Amphibians, such as frogs, breathe through their skin and so they must keep their skin moist, which is why they stay close to water.

Tortoises and turtles
Body armour can help to protect slow moving animals, like tortoises, from attack. The shells of tortoises may be hard, but they can still be damaged.

THE BRAIN AND NERVOUS SYSTEM

The brain coordinates all your body's movements and is active even while you are asleep. The brain is connected to nerves throughout the body by the spinal cord, which runs up your back, protected within your backbone. Information passes very quickly up and down this pathway, to and from the different parts of your body, in the form of electrical impulses.

Saltasaurus

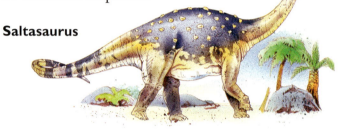

The human brain

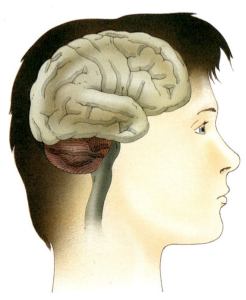

Two-brained dinosaurs
Fossilized sauropod dinosaur remains suggest that these dinosaurs had two small brains. They probably had one brain located above their hind legs plus a small brain in their heads.

The two sides of your brain
The brain controls our bodies. It regulates all our movements and thoughts. The left half of our brain controls the actions of the right side of our body, and the right half of our brain controls the actions of the left side of our body.

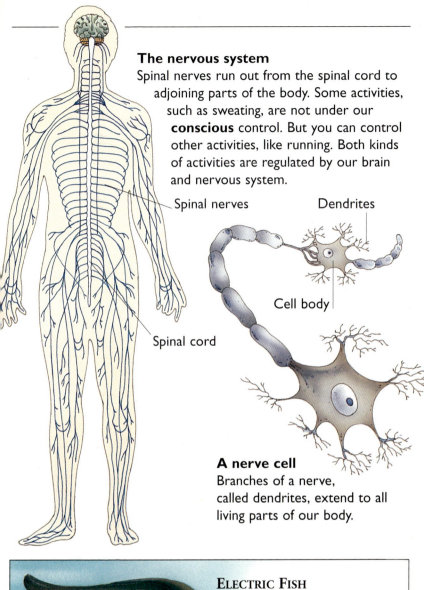

The nervous system
Spinal nerves run out from the spinal cord to adjoining parts of the body. Some activities, such as sweating, are not under our **conscious** control. But you can control other activities, like running. Both kinds of activities are regulated by our brain and nervous system.

Spinal nerves

Dendrites

Cell body

Spinal cord

A nerve cell
Branches of a nerve, called dendrites, extend to all living parts of our body.

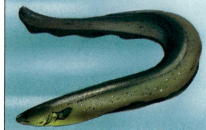

ELECTRIC FISH
Some fish can produce electricity from their nervous systems. The deadly electric eel can generate as much as 650 volts – enough electricity to kill a large animal.

MUSCLES AND NERVES

Muscles control the body's movements. The most active **skeletal muscles** are those controlling the eyes. These move about 100,000 times every day, even when we are asleep.

Most muscles are paired, with the contraction of one muscle extending its opposite partner. They are called antagonistic because one muscle works against the other.

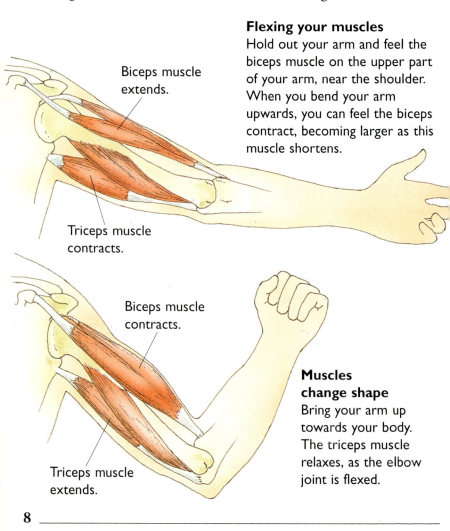

Flexing your muscles
Hold out your arm and feel the biceps muscle on the upper part of your arm, near the shoulder. When you bend your arm upwards, you can feel the biceps contract, becoming larger as this muscle shortens.

Biceps muscle extends.

Triceps muscle contracts.

Biceps muscle contracts.

Muscles change shape
Bring your arm up towards your body. The triceps muscle relaxes, as the elbow joint is flexed.

Triceps muscle extends.

When we want to flex our elbow **joint**, a signal is sent from the cerebral cortex in the brain. This message travels down through the spinal cord and triggers the nerves to the appropriate muscle.

Nerve-muscle interaction
The nerve contains nerve fibres called **axons**, rather like strands of electrical wire encased in plastic.

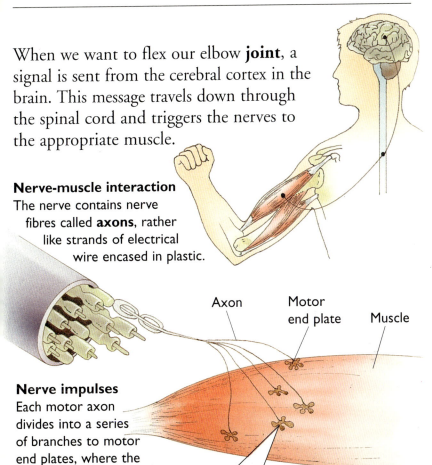

Axon · Motor end plate · Muscle

Nerve impulses
Each motor axon divides into a series of branches to motor end plates, where the nerve meets the muscle.

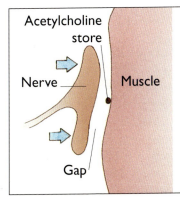

Acetylcholine store · Nerve · Muscle · Gap

THE SYNAPSE
*In the nerves at the motor end plates, there are tiny stores of a chemical transmitter called acetylcholine. This chemical is released by the electrical impulse from the nerve and travels across a gap called a **synapse** to reach the muscle, causing the muscle fibres to contract.*

EYES

Our eyes provide us with our main source of information about the world we live in. All mammals have a pair of eyes set in sockets in the skull, but the position of their eyes varies greatly. Animals, such as rabbits, which are likely to be attacked by other creatures, have their eyes positioned on the sides of their head. This allows them to locate danger easily.

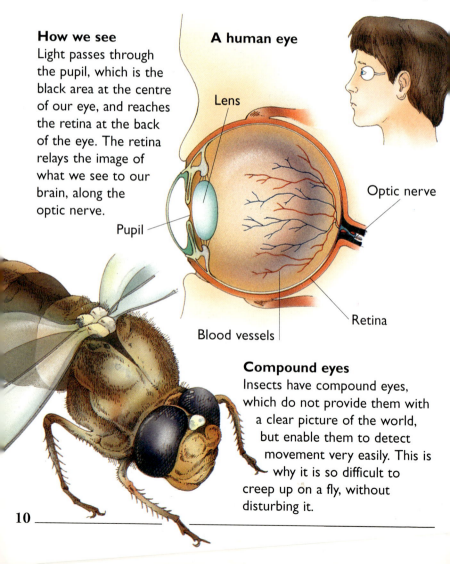

How we see
Light passes through the pupil, which is the black area at the centre of our eye, and reaches the retina at the back of the eye. The retina relays the image of what we see to our brain, along the optic nerve.

A human eye

Lens
Pupil
Optic nerve
Retina
Blood vessels

Compound eyes
Insects have compound eyes, which do not provide them with a clear picture of the world, but enable them to detect movement very easily. This is why it is so difficult to creep up on a fly, without disturbing it.

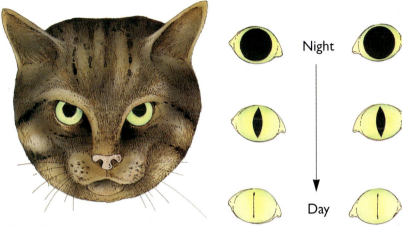

Night

Day

Closely set eyes
Cats and other hunting animals have eyes which point forwards. By superimposing the images from each eye, which overlap slightly, the brain provides the cat with a very accurate picture of the position of its prey.

Colour blindness
Distinguishing features amongst an array of different coloured dots is a good test for colour blindness.

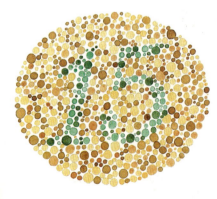

Letting light in
The shape of cats' pupils varies, depending on whether it is sunny or dark. At night the pupils are fully opened, to capture as much light as possible. In bright sunlight they constrict to slit-like openings.

Seeing at night and in colour
The retina, at the back of the eye, contains special cells called rods and cones. While cones are needed for colour vision, animals that hunt at night have more rods in their retinas, because these cells work better when the light is poor. Cats can see objects quite clearly in the dark which would not be visible to us. Not everyone can see individual colours easily. About one in thirty people, mostly men, are unable to distinguish between the colours red and green.

EARS

Our ears are important to us not just for hearing, but also for balance. This is the function of the semi-circular canals in our ears.

How we hear

The ear consists of the outer ear, the middle ear and the inner ear. A sound passes into the outer ear, and reaches the eardrum, causing a vibration which passes into the middle ear. This continues, like an echo, through the ear ossicle bones. The vibrations cause movement in the fluid in the cochlea, in the inner ear. This is then picked up by the auditory nerve, and the sound is carried to the brain.

Earflap

Earflaps

The main purpose of earflaps is to trap sound waves and channel them down into the middle ear. In some mammals, such as the African elephant, the earflaps are very large. An elephant flaps its ears to help it to stay cool.

Ears vary throughout the animal kingdom. Fish do not have ears, but instead, have lateral lines along their bodies to detect sound waves. Birds also have no earflaps but have ear holes, usually hidden by feathers. Marine mammals, like whales and seals, also lack earflaps.

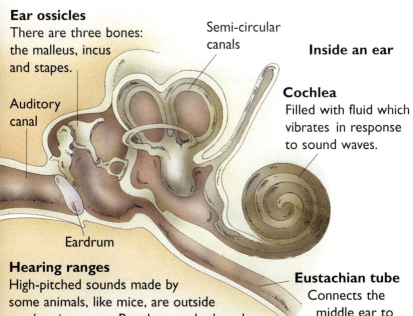

Ear ossicles
There are three bones: the malleus, incus and stapes.

Semi-circular canals

Inside an ear

Auditory canal

Cochlea
Filled with fluid which vibrates in response to sound waves.

Eardrum

Hearing ranges
High-pitched sounds made by some animals, like mice, are outside our hearing range. But they can be heard clearly by other animals, for example, cats.

Eustachian tube
Connects the middle ear to the throat.

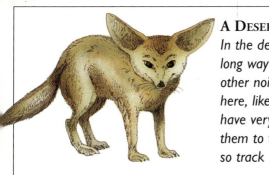

A Desert Fox
In the desert, sounds travel a long way because there is little other noise. Animals which hunt here, like this fennec fox, usually have very large ears. This helps them to trap sound waves and so track down food more easily.

NOSES

The insides of our nostrils are lined with hairs, which act as filters to keep out dust. There are also tiny **glands** in the lining of our nose which produce **mucus**. This traps smaller particles of dust, preventing them from entering our lungs, where they could cause irritation and coughing. Trapped dust particles can be removed by blowing our nose. Air is warmed as it passes up the nostrils, gaining heat from the many blood vessels here.

Cross section of our airways

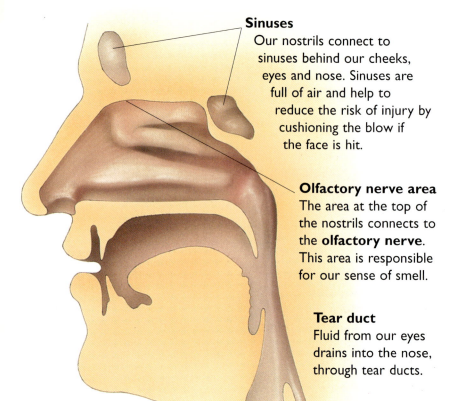

Sinuses
Our nostrils connect to sinuses behind our cheeks, eyes and nose. Sinuses are full of air and help to reduce the risk of injury by cushioning the blow if the face is hit.

Olfactory nerve area
The area at the top of the nostrils connects to the **olfactory nerve**. This area is responsible for our sense of smell.

Tear duct
Fluid from our eyes drains into the nose, through tear ducts.

Windpipe

Elephant's nose

An elephant's nose is joined with its upper lip, forming a trunk. An elephant sucks water up through its nose and squirts it into its mouth when drinking, or over its body if it is taking a shower. An elephant also uses its trunk to pull down branches to eat.

Ivory tusks are actually enlarged teeth.

Dog's nose

The shape of a dog's nose affects its ability to detect scents. Dogs with long, broad noses make the best trackers. Dogs' sense of smell is about one hundred times more sensitive than our own.

Nose looks shiny because it is moist.

Male mandrill

Some animals use their colourful noses to communicate with each other. The male mandrill uses his nose to act as a warning to other males, who might want a fight.

Only adult mandrills have scarlet noses.

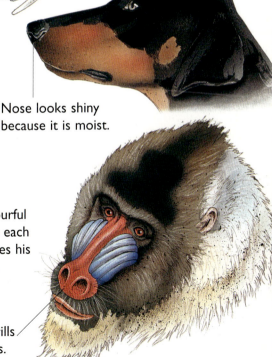

BLOOD AND THE HEART

Our bodies contain about five litres of blood, which consists mainly of red and white blood cells in a fluid called plasma. Red blood cells carry oxygen from the lungs round the body, and bring carbon dioxide back to the lungs. This is made possible by a chemical called **haemoglobin**. Each red blood cell has a life of about three months.

Blood cells
Most blood cells are made in the bone marrow of our bodies. Some white blood cells are produced in the spleen and by lymph nodes round the body.

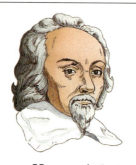

WILLIAM HARVEY (1578-1657)
In 1628 William Harvey proved that blood was circulated round the body, and that the heart was responsible for this movement.

Aorta
Arteries
Heart
Veins

The heart pumps blood round the body. The heart is made up of four chambers – two **atria** and two **ventricles**, separated from each other by valves. As the heart contracts, blood moves from the atria into the ventricles.

The heart

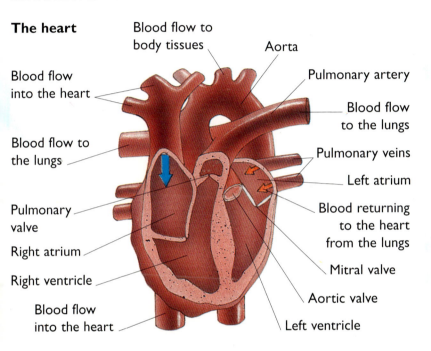

Your pulse

You can measure the rate of your heartbeat by taking your **pulse**. Press on the underside of your wrist. You should feel the movements in the artery wall there, caused by the pumping action of your heart. Count these for a minute, to find out your heart rate – how many times your heart beats per minute.

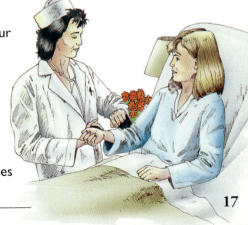

THE FEMALE BODY

Red blood vessels are arteries.
Blue blood vessels are veins.

- Brain
- Carotid artery
- Subclavian artery
- Jugular vein
- Subclavian vein

ANIMAL BODIES

1 Black rhinoceros (Africa)
The pointed upper lip can be used rather like a hand, to pull vegetation. The horns are not made of bone, but keratin – the main component of our hair.

2 Duck-billed platypus (Australia)
This is one of only three living mammals which lay eggs. The duck-like beak helps the platypus to find food underwater, probing through mud for worms and other similar creatures hidden here.

3 Frilled lizard (Australia and Papua New Guinea)
Its bright collar of skin is raised to frighten predators.

4 White's tree frog (Australia and Papua New Guinea)
Sticky sucker pads on the toes of this frog help it to balance on lily leaves and climb trees.

5 Giant anteater (Central and South America)
The anteater's sharp claws help it to crack open the nests of ants and termites, so that its long tongue can probe inside to catch insects.

6 Greater flamingo (Caribbean and Galapagos Islands)
Its bill acts as a filter, sieving out the tiny water creatures which it eats. These creatures contain the coloured pigment which makes the flamingo's plumage pink.

7 Jacana (The Americas)
Very long toes mean this bird can walk easily on thin water lily pads, without sinking into the water.

8 Koala (Australia)
Sharp claws help the koala to climb without falling, and it spends most of its life in the treetops, feeding on eucalyptus leaves.

9 Scarlet-tufted malachite sunbird (Africa)
A long narrow bill allows this bird to probe flowers and find sweet nectar. The sunbird also pollinates flowers when feeding.

10 Tree kangaroo (Australia)
A tree kangaroo has special feet to help it climb and its tail provides balance in the trees where it lives.

11 Pond terrapin (The Americas)
Terrapins live mainly in water. Their shells are flatter in shape than those of tortoises, which helps them to swim fast.

12 White-spotted gecko (Middle East and North Africa)
The large, flat tips of this lizard's toes allow it to run straight up walls, without sliding off. Its colouration can change, to match its background.

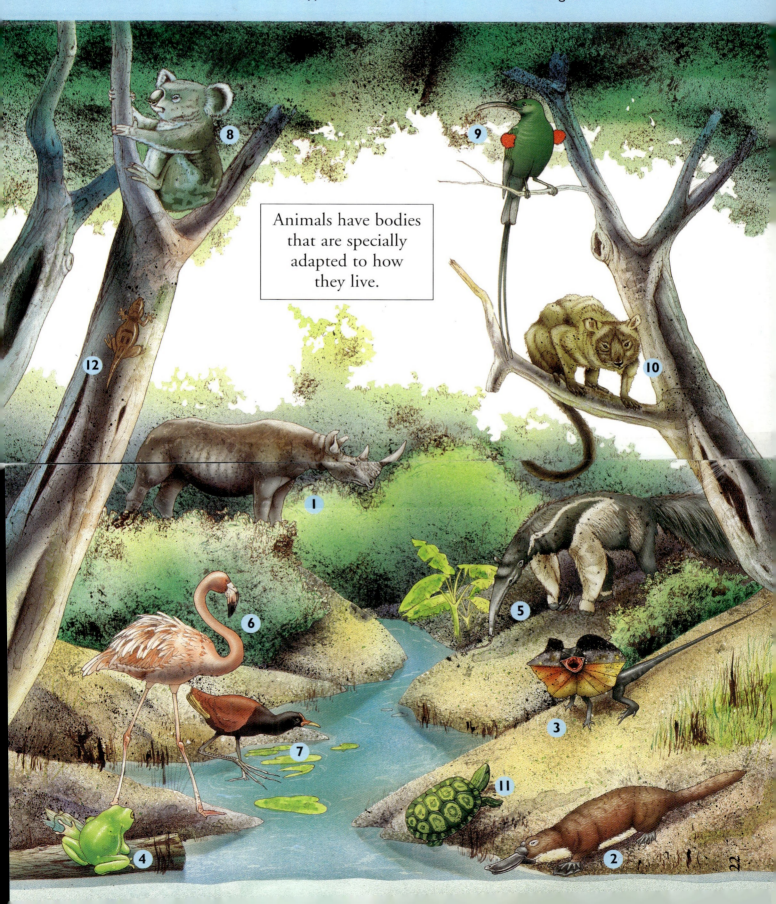

Animals have bodies that are specially adapted to how they live.

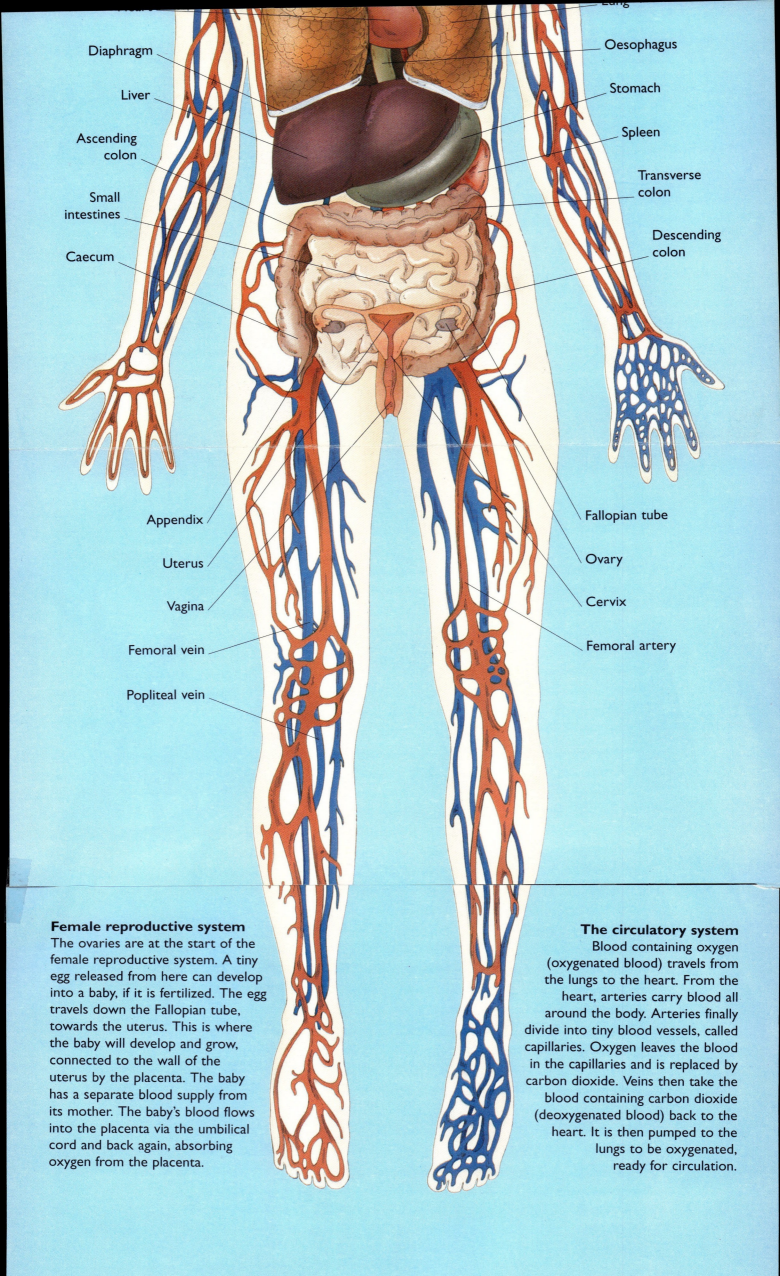

Female reproductive system
The ovaries are at the start of the female reproductive system. A tiny egg released from here can develop into a baby, if it is fertilized. The egg travels down the Fallopian tube, towards the uterus. This is where the baby will develop and grow, connected to the wall of the uterus by the placenta. The baby has a separate blood supply from its mother. The baby's blood flows into the placenta via the umbilical cord and back again, absorbing oxygen from the placenta.

The circulatory system
Blood containing oxygen (oxygenated blood) travels from the lungs to the heart. From the heart, arteries carry blood all around the body. Arteries finally divide into tiny blood vessels, called capillaries. Oxygen leaves the blood in the capillaries and is replaced by carbon dioxide. Veins then take the blood containing carbon dioxide (deoxygenated blood) back to the heart. It is then pumped to the lungs to be oxygenated, ready for circulation.

FINGERS AND TOES

We use our fingers to do all kinds of things, from hanging onto a ladder to picking up delicate objects. This is made possible because of the muscles in our hands. These muscles are linked to **tendons** which control the movements of the joints in our fingers. All our muscles are controlled by nerves.

Gripping
Muscles have to exert exactly the right amount of pressure.

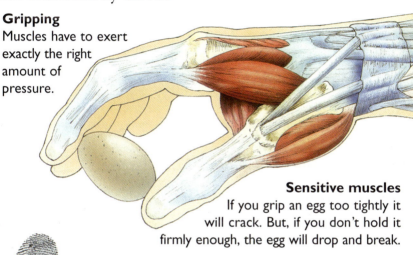

Sensitive muscles
If you grip an egg too tightly it will crack. But, if you don't hold it firmly enough, the egg will drop and break.

Fingerprints
The surface of the skin on our fingers is covered with ridges. These are known as fingerprint patterns. Each person has his or her own unique set of fingerprints.

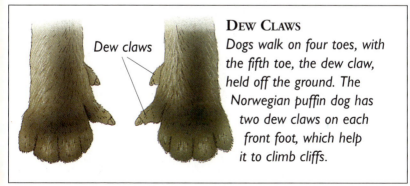

Dew claws

DEW CLAWS
Dogs walk on four toes, with the fifth toe, the dew claw, held off the ground. The Norwegian puffin dog has two dew claws on each front foot, which help it to climb cliffs.

BREATHING

All living cells in our body need oxygen. This gas acts as a fuel, which allows food to be converted into energy. Air containing oxygen is taken into our body when we breathe in through our nose or mouth. The air passes down in a tube, called the windpipe, to the lungs in our chest.

How we breathe

As we inhale, our lungs expand with air. The air passages within the lungs are like a branching tree. Oxygen moves into the bloodstream from tiny branches called the **alveoli**, with carbon dioxide leaving the blood at the same time. When we exhale, the unwanted carbon dioxide passes out.

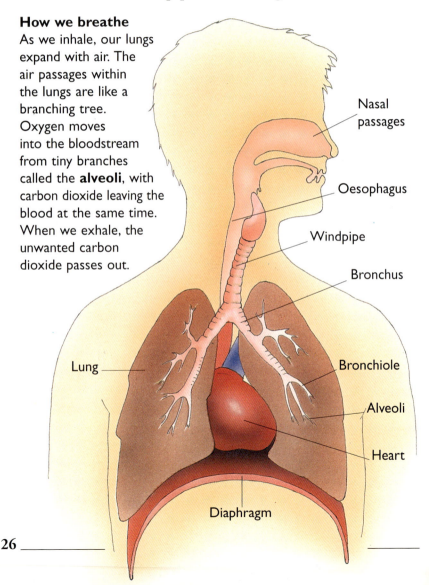

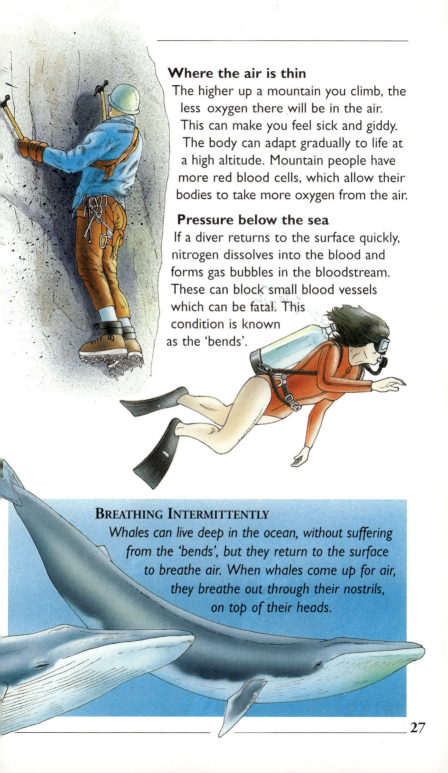

Where the air is thin

The higher up a mountain you climb, the less oxygen there will be in the air. This can make you feel sick and giddy. The body can adapt gradually to life at a high altitude. Mountain people have more red blood cells, which allow their bodies to take more oxygen from the air.

Pressure below the sea

If a diver returns to the surface quickly, nitrogen dissolves into the blood and forms gas bubbles in the bloodstream. These can block small blood vessels which can be fatal. This condition is known as the 'bends'.

BREATHING INTERMITTENTLY

Whales can live deep in the ocean, without suffering from the 'bends', but they return to the surface to breathe air. When whales come up for air, they breathe out through their nostrils, on top of their heads.

TONGUE AND TASTE

Our tongue lies at the bottom of our mouth, and while we can move the front very easily, it is firmly anchored at the back by muscles. Glands in our mouth produce saliva, which keeps our mouth moist. When we eat, more saliva is produced which helps us to soften and swallow our food.

Papillae
These are raised areas on the surface of the tongue, making it feel rough.

Taste buds
These are found in the papillae. There are more than 10,000 taste buds on the human tongue.

Soft palate

Uvula

Bitter tastes detected here.

Salty tastes are sensed here, on both sides.

Sweet items register here, at the tip of the tongue.

Sour tastes are picked up on both sides of our tongue, behind the salt tasting receptors.

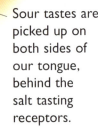

A useful tongue
Cats use their tongues like a ladle, expanding them at the tip to lap up drinks easily. Cats also use their tongues for grooming. Cats' tongues have a rough surface that helps remove dead hairs.

A deceptive tongue
Some animals use their tongues for hunting. The alligator snapping turtle from North America waits for fish to swim into its mouth and then closes its jaws. The fish are lured by the shape of the turtle's tongue, mistaking it for a worm.

A chameleon's tongue
Chameleons are skilled hunters. They have long tongues which can be shot out of the mouth, just like a dart, with great accuracy.

The chameleon's prey sticks to the tip of the tongue, which is then pulled back into its mouth. This all happens so quickly, in just a fraction of a second, that it is hard to see except in slow motion. The muscles in the tongue and a bone at the back of the mouth propel the tongue out of the chameleon's mouth at high speed.

THE DIGESTIVE SYSTEM

We use our teeth to chew food before we swallow it. The narrow incisor and canine teeth at the front of our mouth allow us to bite chunks of food, which are ground down by the molar teeth at the back of our mouth.

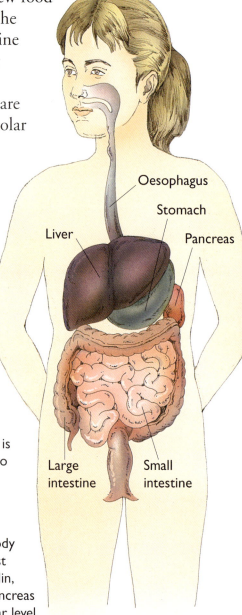

The digestive process
Food passes down the **oesophagus** into the stomach, where it is mixed with digestive juices and ends up as a thickish liquid called chyme. This then passes through the small intestine. Enzymes, which are chemicals that break down food into simple substances, are released from the pancreas into the small intestine. Bile from the gall bladder, which is attached to the liver, helps to break down fatty foods.

Hormones
Hormones are chemical messengers that help the body to function. One of the most important hormones is insulin, which is produced in the pancreas and regulates the body's sugar level.

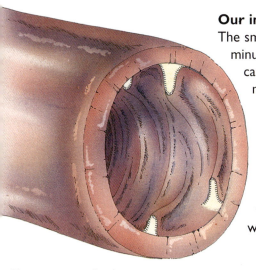

Our intestines

The small intestine is lined with minute finger-like projections called **villi**, through which most of the basic ingredients in food are taken up into the body. After leaving the small intestine, the remains of the food enters the large intestine. Here, water is taken into the body, along with some vitamins.

Four stomachs in one

Cows have a four chambered stomach to help them digest the plants and grasses which they eat. Bacteria help digestion.

Bacteria and tiny organisms called protozoa live in two of a cow's stomach chambers – the rumen and reticulum. When cows are resting, food is regurgitated up into the mouth, chewed and swallowed again.

At the next stage of a cow's digestive process, food passes into another stomach chamber, the omasum. Here, water is absorbed, and food carries on through the abomasum and intestines, to complete the digestive process.

THE URINARY SYSTEM

Our bodies need to remove waste substances. This process is known as excretion. The lungs exhale carbon dioxide, while solid waste is passed out of the intestines. The kidneys have the task of filtering out unwanted nitrogen and other substances from the blood, as well as any excess water. They also help to balance the level of salt in our body.

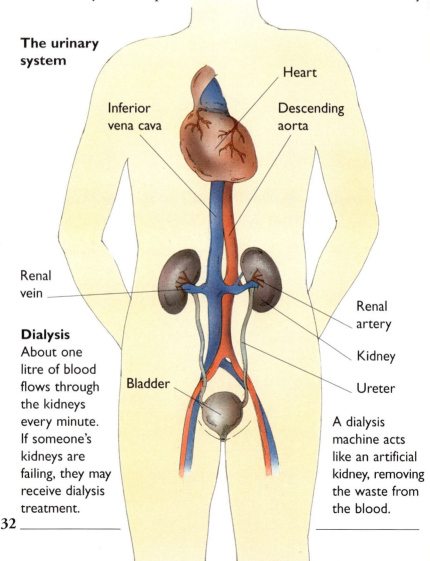

The urinary system

Dialysis
About one litre of blood flows through the kidneys every minute. If someone's kidneys are failing, they may receive dialysis treatment.

A dialysis machine acts like an artificial kidney, removing the waste from the blood.

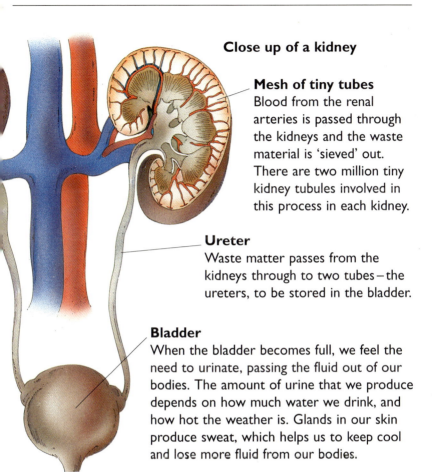

Close up of a kidney

Mesh of tiny tubes
Blood from the renal arteries is passed through the kidneys and the waste material is 'sieved' out. There are two million tiny kidney tubules involved in this process in each kidney.

Ureter
Waste matter passes from the kidneys through to two tubes – the ureters, to be stored in the bladder.

Bladder
When the bladder becomes full, we feel the need to urinate, passing the fluid out of our bodies. The amount of urine that we produce depends on how much water we drink, and how hot the weather is. Glands in our skin produce sweat, which helps us to keep cool and lose more fluid from our bodies.

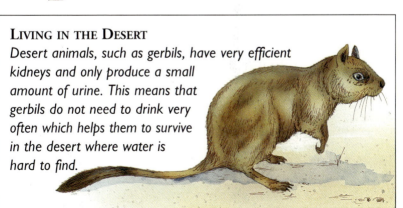

LIVING IN THE DESERT
Desert animals, such as gerbils, have very efficient kidneys and only produce a small amount of urine. This means that gerbils do not need to drink very often which helps them to survive in the desert where water is hard to find.

REPRODUCTION

The mating process results in sperm from the male fertilizing the female's eggs. This is known as reproduction. Whereas birds lay hard-shelled eggs in nests, almost all mammals give birth to live young. Their eggs develop in the part of the female's body called the uterus or womb. The length of time it takes for the young to grow here, up to the stage of being born, is called the **gestation period**.

Hereditary features
Babies often have features of both their parents. Eye and hair colour are two **traits** that are passed on through **genes**.

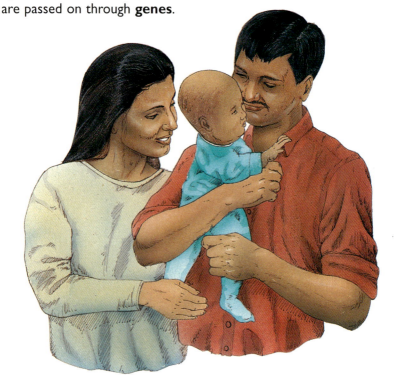

Gestation periods
The female Indian elephant has the longest gestation period of all animals – over two years. Baby elephants are about 90 centimetres tall at birth. A human baby takes nine months to grow inside its mother's body. But we then spend longer caring for our young than any other animal.

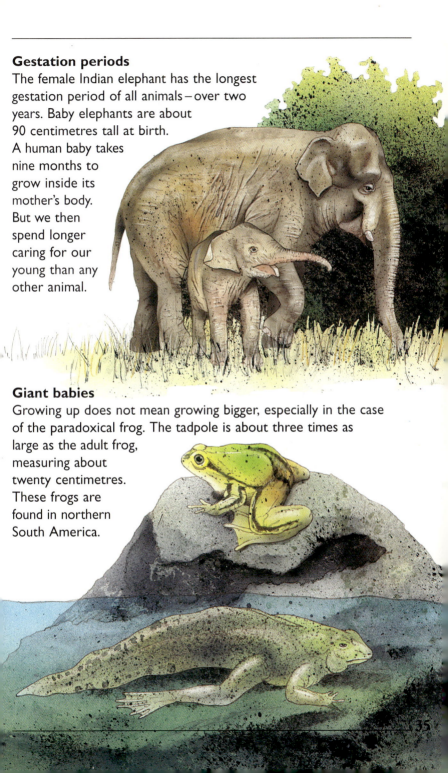

Giant babies
Growing up does not mean growing bigger, especially in the case of the paradoxical frog. The tadpole is about three times as large as the adult frog, measuring about twenty centimetres. These frogs are found in northern South America.

AMAZING BODY FACTS

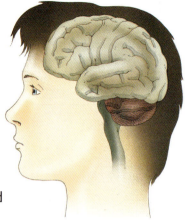

- **Body cells** Cells lining the intestine last just three days, but brain cells can survive throughout our lives.

- **Eyesight** There are over 100 million cells at the back of each eyeball, which enable us to see.

- **Heart power** The heart has the strength to pump a jet of blood two metres high up into the air.

- **Strong creature** The rhinoceros beetle can lift objects that are 850 times its own weight. We can lift objects that are equal to seventeen times our own body weight.

- **Loudest sound** The call of the blue whale can be heard by another whale over 850 kilometres away on the other side of the ocean. Human voices can rarely be heard clearly more than 180 metres away.

- **Muscle power** There are a total of 639 muscles in the human body. These make up about half of our total body weight.

- **Nail growth** Fingernails grow about one millimetre each month, which is four times faster than toenails.

- **Hair** We have about 120,000 hairs on our head. Our hair grows at a rate of about one-and-a-quarter centimetres a month. Hair has been known to grow to almost four metres in length.

- **Sneezing** This can cause particles to be blown out of our nose at a speed of 167 kilometres per hour, which is much faster than the top speed of most cars.

GLOSSARY

Alveoli The smallest airways in the lungs where oxygen passes into the blood, and carbon dioxide leaves it.

Atria The chambers in the heart where blood returns from the body or the lungs.

Axon The connecting nerve fibre running from a nerve cell to a nerve ending.

Conscious Something which we are aware of, or an action which we can control, such as standing up.

Gene Part of the blueprint in our bodies that determines how we look and how our bodies function.

Gestation period The time taken for young mammals to develop in their mothers' bodies, before being born.

Gland An organ in the body, such as the pancreas, which releases chemicals.

Haemoglobin The colour pigment in our blood that makes it appear red, and carries oxygen from the lungs.

Joint The place where two bones join together and movement can take place.

Mucus A substance that keeps surfaces in the body moist, preventing infection or injury.

Oesophagus The tube that connects the mouth to the stomach.

Olfactory nerve The nerve carrying a scent to the brain.

Pulse The movement produced in the arteries by the heart beating.

Skeletal muscle Those muscles in our bodies which allow our skeleton to move.

Synapse The gap between the nerve fibre and the muscle.

Tendon A tough fibrous link which binds skeletal muscles onto bones.

Trait Characteristic, such as hair or eye colour, which is passed from parents to their offspring, through genes.

Ventricles The chambers in the heart which contract to drive blood out into the lungs or the body.

Villi Projections in the small intestine through which nutrients pass into the body.

INDEX *(Entries in **bold** refer to an illustration)*

A
	pages
alligator snapping turtle	29
amphibian	5

B
balance	12, 24
biceps	8
bird	5, 13, 24
bladder	32, 33
blood	16, 17, 26, 27, 32, 33, 37
blood cell	16, 27
brain	6, 7, 9, 10, 11, 12, 36
breathing	26-27

C
carbon dioxide	16, 26, 32, 37
cat	11, 13, 28
chameleon	29
claw	24, 25
colour blindness	11
cow	31

D
desert fox	13
digestive system	30-31
dog	15, 25

E
ear	12-13
egg	21, 24, 25, 34
electric eel	7
elephant	12, 15, 35
excretion	32
eye	10-11, 14, 36

F
	pages
fertilize	21, 34
finger	25
fingerprint	25
fish	5, 13, 29
frog	5, 35

G
gerbil	33
gestation period	34, 35

H
haemoglobin	16, 37
hair	5, 14, 24, 36
Harvey, William	16
heart	16, 17, 19, 21, 26, 32, 36
hedgehog	5

I
intestine	30, 31

J
joint	9, 25

K
kidney	32, 33

L
lip	24
lung	14, 16, 19, 21, 26, 32

M
mammal	5, 10, 13
mandrill	15
mouth	15, 26, 28
muscle	8-9, 25, 28, 29, 36